GROWING

MEDICINAL

HERBS

SOLOMON RICHARDS

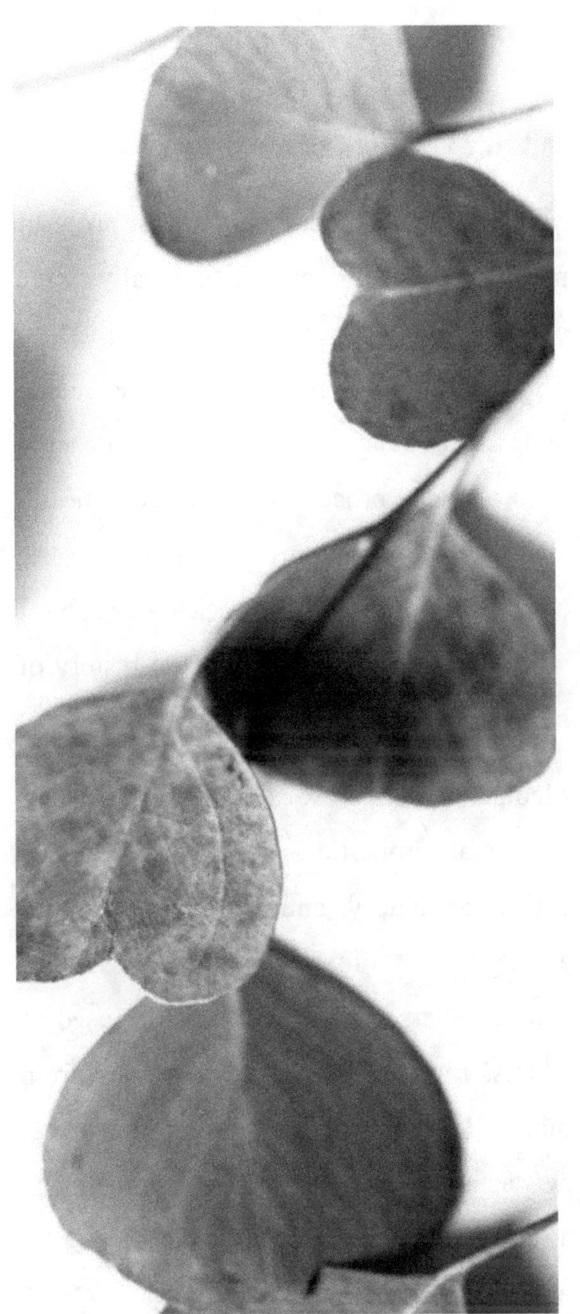

INTRODUCTION

What are Medicinal Herbs?

Medicinal herbs encompass a vast array of plant species that contain biologically active compounds with therapeutic properties. These compounds interact with the human body in various ways, influencing physiological processes to promote health and alleviate symptoms of illness. The use of medicinal herbs dates back thousands of years and is deeply rooted in the history of human civilization.

Medicinal herbs are cultivated for their medicinal properties, which may include anti-inflammatory, antimicrobial, analgesic, antioxidant, and immunomodulatory effects, among others. These herbs can be used to address a wide range of health issues, from minor ailments like indigestion and headaches to more chronic conditions such as arthritis and cardiovascular disease.

The cultivation and utilization of medicinal herbs are not limited to any particular culture or geographic region. Instead, diverse cultures around the world have developed their own herbal traditions based on local plant resources, environmental conditions, and cultural beliefs. This diversity highlights the adaptability and versatility of medicinal herbs as valuable resources for promoting health and well-being.

In addition to their therapeutic benefits, medicinal herbs also play a significant role in culinary traditions, aromatic applications, and spiritual practices. Many herbs are used to enhance the flavor of foods, create fragrant essential oils, or facilitate meditation and relaxation rituals.

Benefits of Growing Medicinal Herbs

1. **Access to Fresh and Potent Remedies**: Growing medicinal herbs allows individuals to access fresh and potent remedies right from their gardens. Freshly harvested herbs retain their maximum potency and nutritional content, ensuring optimal therapeutic benefits.

2. **Customization and Personalization:** By growing medicinal herbs at home, individuals can customize their herbal remedies to suit their specific health needs and preferences. They can experiment with different plant combinations, concentrations, and preparation methods to create personalized formulations tailored to their unique requirements.

3. **Sustainability and Environmental Stewardship**: Cultivating medicinal herbs in home gardens promotes sustainability and environmental stewardship by reducing reliance on commercially grown herbs that may be subject to unsustainable agricultural practices or long-distance transportation. Growing herbs organically also minimizes exposure to harmful pesticides and synthetic fertilizers, protecting both human health and the environment.

4. **Empowerment and Self-Sufficiency:** Growing medicinal herbs empowers individuals to take control of their health and well-being by providing them with the knowledge and resources to care for themselves and their families. It fosters a sense of self-sufficiency and resilience in the face of health challenges, reducing dependence on external healthcare systems and pharmaceutical interventions.

5. **Connection to Nature and Therapeutic Gardening:** Gardening medicinal herbs offers numerous psychological and emotional benefits, including stress reduction, mood enhancement, and increased connection to nature. Engaging in therapeutic gardening activities, such as planting, pruning, and harvesting herbs, can promote relaxation, mindfulness, and a sense of fulfillment.

Importance of Medicinal Herbs in Traditional Medicine

1. **Cultural Heritage and Indigenous Wisdom**: Medicinal herbs are an integral part of traditional medicine systems that have been passed down through generations as a repository of cultural heritage and indigenous wisdom. These ancient healing traditions reflect deep connections to the

natural world and profound respect for the interdependence of all living beings.

2. Holistic Approach to Health and Healing: Traditional medicine systems, such as Ayurveda, Traditional Chinese Medicine (TCM), and Indigenous healing practices, embrace a holistic approach to health and healing that encompasses the physical, emotional, mental, and spiritual dimensions of human existence. Medicinal herbs are viewed as allies in restoring balance and harmony within the body, mind, and spirit.

3. Plant-Driven Therapeutics and Herbal Pharmacopoeias: Traditional medicine systems have developed sophisticated herbal pharmacopoeias based on empirical observations, clinical experience, and ancient texts. These herbal traditions recognize the diverse therapeutic properties of medicinal plants and their potential to treat a wide range of health conditions, from acute infections to chronic diseases.

4. **Complementary and Integrative Medicine:** In recent years, there has been a growing recognition of the value of integrating traditional medicine with conventional healthcare approaches to achieve more comprehensive and patient-centered care. Medicinal herbs play a crucial role as complementary therapies that can enhance the efficacy of conventional treatments, minimize side effects, and promote holistic healing.

5. **Community Health and Resilience**: Traditional medicine practices are often deeply embedded within local communities and serve as sources of resilience and collective well-being. The sharing of herbal

knowledge, remedies, and healing rituals fosters social cohesion, solidarity, and mutual support, contributing to the overall health and resilience of communities in the face of adversity.

Medicinal herbs hold immense cultural, ecological, and therapeutic significance as valuable resources for promoting health, healing, and well-being. By honoring and preserving traditional herbal knowledge, cultivating medicinal herbs sustainably, and integrating herbal medicine into modern healthcare systems, we can harness the full potential of these natural remedies to create healthier, more resilient communities and a more harmonious relationship with the natural world.

CHAPTER ONE

FACTORS TO CONSIDER WHEN GROWING HERBS

Choosing the Right Location

1. **Sunlight Exposure**: Understanding the sunlight exposure needs of medicinal herbs is crucial. Some herbs, like basil and oregano, thrive in full sun, while others, such as ginseng and goldenseal, prefer partial shade. Observing the sun patterns in your garden throughout the day can help you determine the best spots for planting.

2. **Protection from Elements**: Shielding your herbs from harsh elements like strong winds or extreme temperatures is essential for their well-being. Consider planting near structures like fences or buildings that can act as windbreaks or provide partial shade during hot afternoons.

3. **Accessibility:** Convenience plays a significant role in maintaining your herb garden. Ensure that your chosen location is easily accessible for routine tasks like watering, weeding, and harvesting. If your garden is too far from your home, you may be less likely to tend to it regularly.

4. **Space Availability**: Different herbs have varying space requirements. Some, like mint and lemon balm, tend to spread vigorously and may need containment to prevent them from overtaking other plants. Plan your garden layout to accommodate the mature size of each herb and provide ample space between plants for air circulation and ease of maintenance.

5. **Environmental Factors**: Consider environmental factors such as air quality,

pollution, and nearby vegetation. Avoid areas near sources of pollution, like roadsides or industrial areas, as pollutants can negatively impact the quality and safety of your herbs. Additionally, certain herbs may benefit from the proximity of companion plants or suffer from competition with aggressive neighboring species.

Sunlight Requirements

1. **Full Sun**: Herbs that thrive in full sun typically require a minimum of 6 hours of direct sunlight per day. Examples include thyme, sage, and lavender. Planting these herbs in sunny locations ensures robust growth, improved flavor, and higher concentrations of beneficial compounds.

2. **Partial Sun/Shade**: Herbs that prefer partial sun or shade can tolerate less direct

sunlight, usually around 4-6 hours per day. Examples include cilantro, parsley, and chives. Planting these herbs in areas with filtered sunlight or partial shade can help prevent sunburn and reduce water stress during hot summer months.

3. **Indoor Cultivation**: Indoor herb gardens require careful attention to sunlight exposure. Place potted herbs near south-facing windows where they can receive maximum sunlight throughout the day. If natural light is limited, supplement with grow lights specifically designed to mimic the full spectrum of sunlight and promote healthy growth.

4. **Monitoring Sun Exposure**: Regularly monitor the sun exposure in your garden to ensure that your herbs receive adequate light. Observe changes in sun patterns throughout

the seasons and adjust the placement of potted herbs or the layout of your garden beds as needed to optimize sunlight exposure for each plant.

Soil Quality and Drainage

1. **Well-Drained Soil**: Proper soil drainage is essential for preventing waterlogging and root rot. Sandy or loamy soils with good drainage properties are ideal for most herbs. To improve drainage in heavy clay soils, incorporate organic amendments like compost, perlite, or coarse sand to enhance soil structure and porosity.

2. **Soil pH**: The pH level of the soil directly affects nutrient availability and plant growth. Most herbs prefer slightly acidic to neutral soil with a pH range between 6.0 and 7.0. Conduct a soil pH test using a home testing

kit or send a soil sample to a local extension service for analysis. Amend acidic soils with lime to raise pH or elemental sulfur to lower pH as needed to create optimal growing conditions for your herbs.

3. **Organic Matter:** Incorporating organic matter into the soil enriches soil fertility, improves water retention, and enhances soil structure. Compost, aged manure, and leaf mulch are excellent sources of organic matter that supply essential nutrients and beneficial microorganisms to the soil. Apply a 2-3 inch layer of organic mulch around herb plants to conserve soil moisture, suppress weed growth, and regulate soil temperature throughout the growing season.

4. **Mulching:** Mulching is a sustainable gardening practice that provides numerous benefits to herb plants and the soil

ecosystem. Organic mulches like straw, shredded leaves, or pine bark help retain soil moisture, reduce erosion, and promote microbial activity in the soil. Apply mulch around herb plants, leaving a few inches of space around the base of each plant to prevent moisture-related diseases and discourage pest infestations.

Climate Considerations

1. **Hardiness Zone:** Hardiness zones categorize geographic regions based on average annual minimum temperatures to guide gardeners in selecting plants that are well-suited to local climate conditions. Consult the USDA Hardiness Zone Map or a similar resource to identify your specific hardiness zone and choose medicinal herbs that are recommended for your zone.

2. **Temperature Range**: Understanding the temperature requirements of medicinal herbs is essential for successful cultivation. Some herbs, such as rosemary and thyme, thrive in warm climates with mild winters, while others, like echinacea and lemon balm, tolerate colder temperatures and light frosts. Select herbs that are adapted to the temperature range and seasonal variations of your region to ensure optimal growth and productivity.

3. **Frost Dates:** Frost dates mark the beginning and end of the frost-free growing season in your area and help determine the appropriate timing for planting and harvesting herb crops. Start seeds indoors or protect tender herb plants with row covers or cold frames to extend the growing season and minimize frost damage during early spring and late fall. Monitor local weather forecasts and take precautions to safeguard

herbs against unexpected frost events that can occur during transitional periods between seasons.

4. **Microclimates:** Microclimates are localized climate conditions within a garden or landscape that may differ from the surrounding area due to factors such as elevation, exposure to sunlight, and proximity to water bodies. Identify microclimates in your garden, such as sheltered alcoves, sunny slopes, or low-lying valleys, and leverage these unique environments to grow a diverse range of medicinal herbs that thrive under varying temperature and moisture conditions. Experiment with different planting locations and observe how microclimates influence the growth and performance of herb plants throughout the growing season.

By considering these comprehensive factors when selecting a location, understanding sunlight requirements, assessing soil quality and drainage, and evaluating climate considerations, beginner herb growers can establish resilient and productive gardens that support the health and vitality of medicinal herb plants.

Essential Tools and Equipment:

a. **Hand Trowel:** This versatile tool is like a miniature shovel and is perfect for digging small holes for planting seeds or transplanting seedlings. Its compact size makes it easy to maneuver in tight spaces.

b. **Pruning Shears:** Also known as secateurs, pruning shears are designed for trimming and harvesting herbs. They come in various sizes and styles, including bypass and anvil pruners, each suited to different types of cuts.

c. **Garden Gloves:** Protect your hands from blisters, thorns, and dirt while working in the garden. Choose gloves made of durable materials that provide both comfort and protection.

d. **Watering Can or Hose**: Depending on the size of your garden, choose between a watering can for smaller areas or a hose for larger ones. Ensure proper watering to keep your herbs healthy and thriving.

e. **Soil pH Tester:** Understanding your soil's pH level is crucial for growing healthy herbs. Most herbs prefer slightly acidic to neutral soil, so regular testing and adjustments can optimize growing conditions.

f. **Garden Fork:** This tool is essential for breaking up compacted soil, aerating the earth, and incorporating organic matter like compost or fertilizer into the soil. Its sturdy design makes it perfect for heavy-duty gardening tasks.

g. **Shovel:** A garden shovel is indispensable for digging holes, moving soil, and transplanting larger herbs. Choose a shovel with a comfortable handle and a durable blade suited to your gardening needs.

h. **Mulch:** Mulching your herb garden helps retain moisture, suppress weeds, regulate soil temperature, and improve soil structure. Organic mulches like straw, shredded leaves, or wood chips also add nutrients to the soil as they decompose.

i. **Sun Protection Gear:** Don't forget to protect yourself from the sun's harmful rays while gardening. Wear a wide-brimmed hat, apply sunscreen, and opt for lightweight, breathable clothing to stay cool and comfortable outdoors.

Containers vs. In-Ground Beds

a. **Containers:**

- Ideal for small spaces, containers offer flexibility and mobility, allowing you to move your herbs as needed for sunlight or weather conditions.

- Choose pots or containers with drainage holes to prevent waterlogging and ensure proper root aeration.

- Container gardening requires regular watering and fertilizing since soil in pots tends to dry out faster and deplete nutrients more quickly.

- Consider the material of the containers (e.g., terracotta, plastic, or fabric) and their insulating properties to protect herbs from extreme temperatures.

b. **In-Ground Beds:**

- In-ground beds provide ample space for herbs to spread their roots and access nutrients from the soil.

- Proper soil preparation is essential for in-ground gardening, including loosening the soil, removing weeds, and amending with compost or organic matter.

- Mulching in-ground beds helps retain moisture, suppress weeds, and regulate soil temperature, creating optimal growing conditions for herbs.

- Consider factors like soil quality, drainage, and sunlight exposure when selecting a location for your in-ground herb garden.

Irrigation Systems

a. Drip Irrigation: A highly efficient watering system, drip irrigation delivers water directly to the roots of plants, minimizing water waste and reducing the risk of fungal diseases.

- Install drip irrigation lines or tubing along rows or around individual plants, adjusting the flow rate and frequency based on your herbs' water needs.

- Drip irrigation systems can be automated with timers or controlled manually, providing precise watering tailored to your garden's requirements.

b. Soaker Hoses: Similar to drip irrigation, soaker hoses release water slowly and evenly along their length, promoting deep root growth and water conservation.

- Lay soaker hoses on the soil surface or bury them slightly to deliver water directly to the root zone while minimizing evaporation and runoff.

- Soaker hoses are cost-effective and easy to install, making them an excellent choice for herb gardens of all sizes.

c. **Sprinkler Systems**: Ideal for larger herb gardens or areas with uniform plant spacing, sprinkler systems distribute water overhead, covering a wide area with minimal effort.

- Choose sprinkler heads with adjustable spray patterns to customize coverage and minimize water waste.

- Monitor weather conditions and adjust sprinkler settings as needed to prevent overwatering or underwatering your herbs.

d. Hand Watering: While manual watering requires more time and effort, it allows you to closely monitor your herbs' water needs and respond accordingly.

- Use a watering can or hose with a gentle spray nozzle to deliver water directly to the base of plants, avoiding wetting the foliage to reduce the risk of disease.

- Water herbs early in the morning or late in the evening to minimize water loss from evaporation and ensure efficient absorption by the roots.

CHAPTER TWO

SELECTING HERBS FOR YOUR GARDEN

1. **Climate and Growing Conditions**: Different herbs thrive in different climates and growing conditions. Consider the climate of your region and choose herbs that will flourish in your area.

2. **Medicinal Properties:** Identify the medicinal properties you are interested in. Some herbs are known for their calming effects, while others are prized for their ability to boost the immune system or aid digestion.

3. **Space and Garden Layout:** Evaluate the space you have available for gardening. Some herbs, like mint, can spread rapidly

and may require containment, while others, like lavender, grow as compact shrubs.

4. **Sunlight Requirements:** Most herbs prefer full sun, but some can tolerate partial shade. Make sure your garden receives adequate sunlight for the herbs you choose.

5. **Soil Quality**: Consider the quality of your soil and whether it needs any amendments to support herb growth. Some herbs prefer well-draining soil, while others thrive in richer, moisture-retentive soil.

6. **Perennial vs. Annual:** Decide whether you want to plant perennial herbs that come back year after year or annual herbs that need to be replanted each season.

7. **Companion Planting:** Some herbs grow well together and can even help deter pests when planted in close proximity. Consider companion planting to maximize the health and yield of your garden.

8. **Availability and Accessibility:** Choose herbs that are readily available in your area or can be easily sourced from nurseries or seed catalogs.

EASY-TO-GROW MEDICINAL HERBS FOR BEGINNERS

1. **Peppermint:** Peppermint is a hardy perennial herb that spreads rapidly. It thrives in rich, moist soil and partial shade.

2. **Lemon Balm**: Lemon balm is another hardy perennial with a delightful lemon

scent. It prefers well-drained soil and partial shade.

3. **Chamomile:** Chamomile is an annual herb that grows easily from seed. It prefers full sun and well-drained soil.

4. **Lavender:** Lavender is a beautiful perennial herb known for its fragrant flowers. It thrives in sunny, well-drained locations.

5. **Calendula:** Calendula is an annual herb with cheerful orange or yellow flowers. It grows well in full sun and tolerates a variety of soil conditions.

6. **Echinacea:** Echinacea is a perennial herb prized for its immune-boosting properties. It prefers full sun and well-drained soil.

7. **Thyme:** Thyme is a low-growing perennial herb that adds flavor to culinary dishes. It thrives in sunny locations with well-drained soil.

Understanding Herb Growth Habits

1. Annuals: Annual herbs complete their life cycle within one growing season. They grow from seed, produce flowers and seeds, and then die back. Examples include basil, cilantro, and chamomile.

2. Perennials: Perennial herbs live for multiple growing seasons, often returning year after year. They may die back in the winter and regrow in the spring. Examples include lavender, thyme, and sage.

3. Biennials: Biennial herbs have a two-year life cycle. They typically grow foliage

during the first year and produce flowers and seeds during the second year before dying back. Examples include parsley and angelica.

4. Herbaceous vs. Woody: Herbaceous herbs have soft, non-woody stems and usually die back in the winter. Woody herbs have woody stems and may remain evergreen or semi-evergreen throughout the year. Examples of herbaceous herbs include basil and cilantro, while examples of woody herbs include rosemary and thyme.

How To Grow Medicinal Herbs for Beginners

Soil Preparation and Planting

Soil Preparation and Planting are fundamental steps in establishing a successful medicinal herb garden.

1. Soil Preparation:

Soil preparation is the foundation of a thriving medicinal herb garden. Before planting, it's essential to assess the soil quality and make necessary amendments to ensure it is fertile, well-draining, and rich in nutrients. The following steps are involved in soil preparation:

- Soil Testing: Conduct soil tests to determine pH levels, nutrient content, and texture. This information guides the selection of appropriate amendments.

- Weed Removal: Remove any existing weeds or debris from the planting area to prevent competition for nutrients and space.

- Tilling or Turning the Soil: Loosen the soil to improve aeration and drainage. This helps plant roots penetrate easily and promotes healthy growth.

2. Soil Amendments:

Soil amendments are substances added to the soil to improve its structure, fertility, and nutrient content. Common soil amendments include:

- Compost: Rich in organic matter, compost enhances soil fertility, promotes beneficial microbial activity, and improves moisture retention.

- Manure: Well-aged animal manure provides essential nutrients such as nitrogen, phosphorus, and potassium, contributing to healthy plant growth.

- Organic Matter: Incorporating organic matter such as leaf mold, peat moss, or shredded bark improves soil structure, increases nutrient availability, and enhances water retention.

- Mineral Amendments: Depending on soil test results, minerals like lime (to raise pH) or sulfur (to lower pH) may be added to adjust soil acidity levels.

3. Plant Spacing and Arrangement:

Proper plant spacing and arrangement are crucial for maximizing sunlight exposure, airflow, and overall plant health. Consider the following factors when planning plant spacing and arrangement:

- Sunlight Requirements: Place taller herbs or those requiring full sun towards the back of the garden to prevent shading of shorter plants.

- Air Circulation: Avoid overcrowding plants to prevent moisture buildup and reduce the risk of fungal diseases.

- Companion Planting: Some medicinal herbs thrive when planted alongside compatible companions that provide pest control, attract beneficial insects, or improve soil health.

- Harvesting Accessibility: Arrange plants in a way that facilitates easy access for harvesting and maintenance tasks.

Weed and Pest Management Strategies

Understanding Weed Management:

Weeds are unwanted plants that compete with medicinal herbs for resources like sunlight, water, and nutrients. Effective weed management is essential for maintaining the health and productivity of your herb garden.

- Mulching: Mulching involves covering the soil around your medicinal herbs with materials like straw, wood chips, or compost. Mulch suppresses weed growth by blocking sunlight and preventing weed seeds from germinating. Additionally, organic mulches decompose over time, enriching the soil with nutrients and improving its structure.

- Hand weeding: Hand weeding is the manual removal of weeds by pulling them out from the root. This method allows you to target specific weeds while minimizing damage to your medicinal herbs. Regularly inspecting your garden and promptly removing weeds can prevent them from spreading and competing with your plants.

- Weed barriers: Weed barriers, such as landscape fabric or cardboard, create a physical barrier between the soil and weed seeds. By preventing weed seeds from coming into contact with the soil, weed barriers inhibit weed germination and growth. Combine weed barriers with organic mulch for optimal weed suppression.

Pest Management Strategies:

Pests, including insects, rodents, and pathogens, pose a threat to the health and yield of medicinal herbs. Implementing effective pest management strategies is essential for preventing pest damage and maintaining the quality of your herbs. :

- Integrated Pest Management (IPM): IPM is a holistic approach to pest management that emphasizes prevention, monitoring, and intervention. It involves regular monitoring of pest populations, identification of pest species, and the use of multiple control methods, including cultural, biological, and chemical controls. By integrating various strategies, such as crop rotation, habitat manipulation, and biological control agents, IPM minimizes the reliance on chemical pesticides and promotes long-term pest control.

- Natural Predators: Introducing beneficial insects, such as ladybugs, lacewings, and parasitic wasps, can help control pest populations naturally. These insects prey on common garden pests like aphids, caterpillars, and mites, reducing the need for chemical interventions. Encouraging biodiversity in your garden by providing habitat and food sources for beneficial insects enhances natural pest control mechanisms.

- Organic Insecticides: In addition to natural predators, organic insecticides derived from plant-based ingredients, such as neem oil, pyrethrin, and insecticidal soap, can effectively manage pest infestations without harming beneficial insects or compromising environmental safety. Organic insecticides disrupt pests' life cycles, repel them from plants, or directly target their physiological processes, providing targeted pest control while minimizing adverse effects on non-target organisms.

In the subsequent chapters, we will explore natural pest control methods and companion planting techniques in greater detail to help you establish a balanced and resilient ecosystem in your medicinal herb garden.

PRUNING AND HARVESTING TECHNIQUES

Timing and Frequency

- Pruning: The timing and frequency of pruning depend on the growth habits of the herb. For instance, perennial herbs like lavender and rosemary benefit from regular pruning to stimulate new growth and maintain their shape. Annual herbs such as basil may need more frequent pruning to prevent them from flowering too early and ensure continued leaf production.

- Harvesting: The timing of harvesting varies depending on the part of the plant you intend to use. For instance, for leafy herbs like mint and cilantro, it's best to harvest leaves when they are young and tender before they become tough and bitter. For herbs like chamomile and calendula, harvesting flowers should ideally occur when they are fully open but before they start to wilt.

Techniques and Tools:

- Pruning: Different pruning techniques include pinching, where you remove the growing tip of the stem to encourage branching, and thinning, where you selectively remove excess growth to improve airflow and light penetration.

- Harvesting: Use sharp scissors or pruning shears to make clean cuts when harvesting herbs. Avoid tearing or bruising the plant, as this can lead to damage and reduce the quality of the harvest.

Considerations:

- Pruning: Consider the overall health and vigor of the plant when deciding on pruning techniques. Remove dead or diseased branches promptly to prevent the spread of pathogens throughout the plant.

- Harvesting: Consider factors such as weather conditions and plant hydration when harvesting herbs. It's best to harvest herbs early in the morning when they are most hydrated and before the heat of the day causes moisture loss.

Understanding Growth Cycles

Germination and Seedling Care:

- Provide adequate moisture and warmth for seeds to germinate successfully. Seedlings require consistent watering and protection from extreme temperatures and pests during their early stages of growth.

- Consider using seedling trays or starting seeds indoors to provide optimal conditions for germination and seedling development.

Vegetative Growth and Nutrient Requirements

- During the vegetative growth stage, herbs require ample sunlight and nutrients to develop strong stems and lush foliage. Consider using organic fertilizers or compost to provide essential nutrients without the risk of chemical buildup.

- Monitor soil moisture levels and adjust watering frequency as needed to prevent overwatering or underwatering, which can stunt growth or lead to root rot.

Flowering and Reproduction:

- Flowering signals a transition from vegetative growth to reproductive growth. Some herbs, like basil and cilantro, may bolt and flower prematurely if they experience stress or prolonged exposure to high temperatures.

- Encourage continuous flowering by deadheading spent flowers regularly and providing optimal growing conditions for the plant.

Dormancy and Overwintering

- Many perennial herbs enter a period of dormancy during the winter months, where growth slows or halts altogether. Prepare herbs for dormancy by gradually reducing watering and fertilizer applications as temperatures drop.

- Consider providing protective mulch or covering for tender herbs to insulate them from freezing temperatures and frost damage.

Harvesting Herbs for Maximum Potency

Understanding Active Compounds:

- Research the active compounds present in the herbs you are growing and understand how they contribute to their medicinal properties. For example, mint contains menthol, which has analgesic and anti-inflammatory effects, while chamomile contains chamazulene, which has soothing and anti-anxiety properties.

Optimal Harvesting Conditions:

- Harvest herbs when their essential oil content is at its peak, which often occurs during the early morning when temperatures are cooler and humidity levels are higher.

- Consider environmental factors such as air quality and pollution levels, as these can affect the potency and purity of harvested herbs.

Drying and Storage Techniques:

- Properly dry harvested herbs to preserve their potency and prevent mold or degradation. Hang herbs upside down in a dry, well-ventilated area away from direct sunlight.

- Store dried herbs in airtight containers in a cool, dark place to protect them from moisture and light exposure, which can degrade their potency over time.

Testing and Quality Assurance:

- Consider investing in testing equipment or working with a reputable laboratory to analyze the potency and purity of harvested herbs. Conducting regular quality assurance checks can help ensure that your herbs meet the highest standards for medicinal use.

Growing Disease Prevention and Management

In the realm of herb cultivation, diseases pose significant threats to plant health and overall yield. Understanding the common herb diseases, along with implementing effective preventative measures and treatment options, is paramount for successful herb cultivation and management. Now we dive into the intricacies of common herb diseases, offering insights into preventative strategies and treatment protocols.

Common Herb Diseases

1. **Powdery Mildew**: Powdery mildew is a fungal disease that affects a wide range of herbs, including basil, rosemary, and oregano. It appears as a white, powdery substance on the leaves, stems, and flowers, inhibiting photosynthesis and weakening the plant.

2. **Downy Mildew**: Downy mildew is another fungal disease that commonly affects herbs such as basil and mint. It manifests as yellow or brown spots on the upper surface of leaves, accompanied by a downy growth on the undersides. Downy mildew can quickly spread and devastate herb crops if not addressed promptly.

3. **Fusarium Wilt**: Fusarium wilt is a soil-borne fungal disease that affects the vascular system of herbs like cilantro, parsley, and dill. It causes wilting, yellowing, and eventual death of the plant by obstructing water and nutrient uptake.

4. **Root Rot**: Root rot is caused by various fungi, including Pythium and Phytophthora, and it affects the root system of herbs, leading to stunted growth, wilting, and plant

death. Overwatering and poor drainage contribute to the development of root rot.

5. **Bacterial Leaf Spot**: Bacterial leaf spot is a bacterial disease characterized by dark, water-soaked lesions on herb leaves. It affects herbs like basil, thyme, and sage, leading to defoliation and reduced yield.

Preventative Measures

1. **Cultural Practices**: Implementing proper cultural practices such as crop rotation, maintaining adequate spacing between plants, and ensuring good air circulation can help prevent the spread of diseases by reducing favorable conditions for pathogens.

2. **Sanitation**: Regularly clean and sanitize gardening tools, pots, and equipment to

prevent the introduction and spread of pathogens. Remove and dispose of infected plant debris to prevent the recurrence of diseases in subsequent growing seasons.

3. **Water Management**: Avoid overwatering herbs, as excessive moisture creates a conducive environment for fungal diseases like powdery mildew and root rot. Water herbs at the base of the plant in the morning to allow foliage to dry before evening, minimizing the risk of disease development.

4. **Resistant Varieties**: Select herb varieties that are resistant to common diseases prevalent in your region. Resistant varieties have genetic traits that enable them to withstand and tolerate disease pressure better than susceptible varieties.

Treatment Options

1. **Fungicides**: Apply fungicides containing active ingredients such as sulfur, copper, or

neem oil to control fungal diseases like powdery mildew and downy mildew. Follow label instructions carefully and apply fungicides during the early stages of disease development for optimal efficacy.

2. **Biological Controls:** Utilize biological control agents such as beneficial fungi and bacteria to suppress the growth and spread of pathogens. Biological controls offer environmentally friendly solutions to managing herb diseases while minimizing the use of synthetic chemicals.

3. **Pruning:** Prune and remove infected plant parts to prevent the spread of diseases within the herb garden. Pruning encourages air circulation and sunlight penetration, creating unfavorable conditions for pathogen proliferation.

4. **Soil Amendments**: Incorporate organic matter and compost into the soil to improve its structure and enhance beneficial microbial activity. Healthy soil promotes strong root development and increases herb resistance to diseases like Fusarium wilt and root rot.

Effective disease prevention and management strategies are essential for maintaining healthy herb crops and ensuring a bountiful harvest. By familiarizing yourself with common herb diseases, implementing preventative measures, and utilizing appropriate treatment options, you can safeguard your herb garden against the detrimental effects of diseases and enjoy thriving plant growth and productivity.

CHAPTER THREE

Understanding Herbal Preparations

Infusions:

Infusions are herbal preparations where hot water is poured over plant materials such as leaves, flowers, or herbs to extract their medicinal properties. The process involves steeping the plant material in hot water for a certain period, allowing the water to absorb the active compounds present in the herbs. Infusions are commonly used for delicate plant parts and are effective for extracting volatile oils, vitamins, and other water-soluble constituents. Temperature, steeping time, and the ratio of herb to water all influence the strength and efficacy of the infusion.

Decoctions:

Decoctions are similar to infusions but are used for tougher plant parts such as roots, bark, and seeds. Unlike infusions, which involve steeping, decoctions require boiling the plant material in water for a longer period. Boiling helps break down the tougher plant fibers and release the medicinal compounds contained within. Decoctions are ideal for extracting alkaloids, bitter principles, and other constituents that are not easily soluble in cold water. The simmering process may vary in duration depending on the hardness of the plant material and the desired strength of the decoction.

 Tinctures:

Tinctures are concentrated herbal extracts made by soaking plant material in alcohol or another solvent. The alcohol acts as a menstruum, extracting both water-soluble and alcohol-soluble compounds from the herbs. Tinctures are known for their potency and long shelf life. They are commonly used when a stronger concentration of medicinal compounds is desired or when the herb's properties are best extracted in alcohol. The ratio of herb to alcohol, as well as the duration of extraction, determines the strength and effectiveness of the tincture.

Simple Herbal Recipes for Beginners

Herbal Tea Blends:

Herbal teas are popular for their soothing and medicinal properties. Simple herbal tea blends can be created using a variety of herbs such as chamomile, peppermint, lemon balm, and ginger. These blends can address various health concerns such as relaxation, digestion, immune support, and respiratory health. Brewing herbal teas involves steeping the herbs in hot water for a certain period, allowing the water to absorb the beneficial compounds present in the herbs.

Healing Salves and Balms:

Healing salves and balms are topical herbal preparations used to soothe skin irritations, minor cuts, burns, and muscle soreness. They are made by infusing herbs such as calendula, comfrey, lavender, or plantain into carrier oils such as olive oil or coconut oil. The infused oil is then mixed with beeswax to create a solid consistency. These herbal preparations provide topical relief and promote healing by reducing inflammation, soothing discomfort, and supporting skin regeneration.

Herbal Syrups and Elixirs:

Herbal syrups and elixirs are sweetened preparations used for immune support, respiratory health, and overall well-being. They are made by combining herbal infusions or decoctions with honey, glycerin, or other sweeteners. Common herbs used in syrups and elixirs include elderberry, echinacea, thyme, and licorice root. These preparations are often taken orally and can be especially beneficial during cold and flu season for boosting the immune system and soothing coughs and sore throats.

Herbal Bath Blends:

Herbal baths offer a relaxing and therapeutic experience by combining the healing properties of herbs with the soothing effects of warm water. Herbal bath blends can include a variety of herbs such as rose petals, lavender buds, chamomile flowers, and oatmeal. These herbs are placed in a muslin bag or directly into the bathwater, allowing their beneficial compounds to infuse into the water. Herbal baths help alleviate stress, promote relaxation, soothe muscle tension, and nourish the skin.

Profiles of Popular Medicinal Herbs

1. Ginseng (Panax ginseng):

- Properties: Ginseng is an adaptogenic herb, meaning it helps the body cope with stress and maintain balance. It's known for its immune-boosting, energy-enhancing, and cognitive function-improving properties.

- Traditional Use: Traditional Chinese Medicine (TCM) has used ginseng for thousands of years to improve vitality, cognitive function, and overall health.

- Modern Applications: Ginseng is commonly used as a tonic for fatigue, to enhance athletic performance, improve mental clarity, and support the immune system.

2. **Turmeric (Curcuma longa):**

- Properties: Turmeric contains curcumin, a compound known for its anti-inflammatory, antioxidant, and anti-cancer properties. It supports joint health, digestion, and liver function.

- Traditional Use: Turmeric has been used for centuries in Ayurvedic medicine to treat various ailments, including arthritis, digestive issues, and skin conditions.

- Modern Applications: Turmeric is widely used as a dietary supplement for its anti-inflammatory benefits, particularly in managing conditions like arthritis, inflammatory bowel disease, and metabolic syndrome.

3. **Echinacea (Echinacea purpurea):**

- Properties: Echinacea is known for its immune-stimulating properties, helping the body fight off infections, especially respiratory infections like the common cold and flu.

- Traditional Use: Native American tribes used echinacea for centuries to treat wounds, infections, and as a general health tonic.

- Modern Applications: Echinacea is commonly used as a preventative measure against colds and flu, and it may also help reduce the severity and duration of symptoms when taken at the onset of illness.

4. Ginkgo (Ginkgo biloba):

- Properties: Ginkgo is renowned for its cognitive-enhancing properties, improving memory, concentration, and overall cognitive function. It also has antioxidant and anti-inflammatory effects.

- Traditional Use: Ginkgo has been used in traditional Chinese medicine for thousands of years to improve blood circulation and cognitive function.

- Modern Applications: Ginkgo is often used to support cognitive health, particularly in older adults experiencing age-related cognitive decline. It may also help improve symptoms of conditions like Alzheimer's disease and vascular dementia.

5. St. John's Wort (Hypericum perforatum):

- Properties: St. John's Wort is primarily known for its antidepressant properties, as it helps regulate mood and alleviate symptoms of mild to moderate depression. It also has anti-inflammatory and wound-healing properties.

- Traditional Use: St. John's Wort has a long history of use in European traditional medicine for treating various ailments, including depression, anxiety, and nerve pain.

- Modern Applications: St. John's Wort is commonly used as a natural remedy for depression, although its effectiveness varies. It may also be used topically to promote wound healing.

6. **Garlic (Allium sativum)**:

- Properties: Garlic is well-known for its antimicrobial, antiviral, and immune-boosting properties. It also has cardiovascular benefits, including lowering blood pressure and cholesterol levels.

- Traditional Use: Garlic has been used for thousands of years in various cultures for its medicinal properties, including its ability to fight infections and promote overall health.

- Modern Applications: Garlic supplements are commonly used to support immune function, cardiovascular health, and to lower the risk of certain infections.

7. Ginger (Zingiber officinale):

- Properties: Ginger is valued for its anti-inflammatory, digestive, and anti-nausea properties. It contains bioactive compounds such as gingerol and shogaol, which contribute to its medicinal effects.

- Traditional Use: Ginger has been used in traditional medicine systems like Ayurveda and Traditional Chinese Medicine to alleviate digestive issues, reduce inflammation, and relieve nausea.

- Modern Applications: Ginger is used to alleviate nausea, motion sickness, and morning sickness during pregnancy. It's also used to relieve pain and inflammation associated with conditions like osteoarthritis and menstrual cramps.

8. **Valerian (Valeriana officinalis):**

- Properties: Valerian is known for its sedative and anxiolytic (anxiety-reducing) properties. It helps promote relaxation and improve sleep quality.

- Traditional Use: Valerian has been used in traditional medicine for centuries as a natural remedy for insomnia, anxiety, and nervous restlessness.

- Modern Applications: Valerian supplements are commonly used as a natural sleep aid and to reduce symptoms of anxiety and stress. It's often used in combination with other herbs like passionflower and lemon balm for enhanced effects.

9. **Chamomile (Matricaria chamomilla):**

- Properties: Chamomile has calming, anti-inflammatory, and antioxidant properties. It's often used to promote relaxation, improve sleep quality, and soothe digestive issues.

- Traditional Use: Chamomile has a long history of use in traditional medicine for its calming effects on the mind and body. It's commonly consumed as a tea to promote relaxation and alleviate digestive discomfort.

- Modern Applications: Chamomile tea is popular for its calming effects and is used to relieve anxiety, stress, and insomnia. It's also used topically in skincare products for its anti-inflammatory and soothing properties.

10. Peppermint (Mentha piperita):

- Properties: Peppermint is known for its digestive benefits, including relieving indigestion, bloating, and nausea. It also has analgesic and antimicrobial properties.

- Traditional Use: Peppermint has been used for centuries in traditional medicine to alleviate digestive issues and soothe respiratory symptoms.

- Modern Applications: Peppermint oil is used to alleviate symptoms of irritable bowel syndrome (IBS), including abdominal pain and bloating. It's also used topically to relieve headaches and muscle pain.

11. Lavender (Lavandula angustifolia):

- Properties: Lavender has calming and sedative properties, making it useful for promoting relaxation, reducing anxiety, and improving sleep quality. It also has anti-inflammatory and analgesic effects.

- Traditional Use: Lavender has been used in herbal medicine for its calming effects on the nervous system and its ability to promote relaxation and improve sleep.

- Modern Applications: Lavender essential oil is used in aromatherapy to reduce anxiety and stress, promote relaxation, and improve sleep quality. It's also used topically to soothe skin irritations and promote wound healing.

12. Aloe Vera (Aloe barbadensis):

- Properties: Aloe vera has anti-inflammatory, antimicrobial, and wound-healing properties. It's commonly used to soothe sunburns, promote wound healing, and moisturize the skin.

- Traditional Use: Aloe vera has been used for centuries in traditional medicine for its medicinal properties, including its ability to heal wounds, soothe skin irritations, and promote digestive health.

- Modern Applications: Aloe vera gel is used topically to soothe sunburns, insect bites, and various skin irritations. It's also used orally as a natural remedy for digestive issues like constipation and irritable bowel syndrome (IBS).

13. **Ashwagandha (Withania somnifera)**:

- Properties: Ashwagandha is an adaptogenic herb known for its stress-relieving, immune-enhancing, and rejuvenating properties. It helps the body cope with stress and promotes overall vitality.

- Traditional Use: Ashwagandha has been used for centuries in Ayurvedic medicine to increase energy, improve cognitive function, and enhance overall health and longevity.

- Modern Applications: Ashwagandha supplements are commonly used to reduce stress, anxiety, and fatigue. It's also used to support adrenal health, improve sleep quality, and enhance athletic performance.

14. **Holy Basil (Ocimum sanctum):**

- Properties: Holy Basil, also known as Tulsi, is revered in Ayurvedic medicine for its adaptogenic, antioxidant, and anti-inflammatory properties. It helps reduce stress, support the immune system, and promote overall well-being.

- Traditional Use: Holy Basil has been used for thousands of years in Ayurveda as a sacred herb to promote longevity, enhance spiritual growth, and alleviate various ailments.

- Modern Applications: Holy Basil supplements are used to reduce stress, promote mental clarity, and support immune function. It's also consumed as a tea for its calming and rejuvenating effects.

15. **Milk Thistle (Silybum marianum):**

- Properties: Milk Thistle contains active compounds like silymarin, known for their hepatoprotective (liver-protective) properties. It supports liver health, detoxification, and regeneration.

- Traditional Use: Milk Thistle has been used in traditional herbal medicine, particularly in Europe, to treat liver disorders, including hepatitis, cirrhosis, and fatty liver disease.

- Modern Applications: Milk Thistle supplements are commonly used to support liver health, especially in individuals with liver conditions or those exposed to toxins. It's also used as a natural remedy for indigestion and gallbladder issues.

16. **Black Cohosh (Actaea racemosa)**:

- Properties: Black Cohosh is known for its hormone-balancing properties, particularly in women. It's used to alleviate symptoms of menopause, including hot flashes, mood swings, and sleep disturbances.

- Traditional Use: Native American tribes used Black Cohosh for centuries to treat various women's health issues, including menstrual irregularities and menopausal symptoms.

- Modern Applications: Black Cohosh supplements are commonly used to relieve symptoms of menopause, such as hot flashes, night sweats, and vaginal dryness. It's also used to regulate menstrual cycles and alleviate symptoms of premenstrual syndrome (PMS).

17. **Saw Palmetto (Serenoa repens):**

- Properties: Saw Palmetto is known for its prostate-supporting properties. It helps reduce symptoms of benign prostatic hyperplasia (BPH), including urinary frequency, urgency, and nocturia.

- Traditional Use: Native Americans used Saw Palmetto berries for centuries to support urinary and reproductive health. It was also used to treat conditions like urinary tract infections and low libido.

- Modern Applications: Saw Palmetto supplements are commonly used by men to alleviate symptoms of BPH and support prostate health. It may also help improve urinary function and reduce inflammation in the urinary tract.

18. **Nettle (Urtica dioica):**

- Properties: Nettle has anti-inflammatory, diuretic, and immune-modulating properties.

It's used to alleviate symptoms of allergies, arthritis, and urinary tract infections.

- Traditional Use: Nettle has been used in traditional medicine for its medicinal properties, including its ability to relieve joint pain, reduce allergy symptoms, and promote urinary tract health.

- Modern Applications: Nettle supplements are commonly used to reduce symptoms of allergic rhinitis (hay fever), including sneezing, runny nose, and itching. It's also used to relieve symptoms of osteoarthritis and support urinary tract health.

19. **Licorice Root (Glycyrrhiza glabra)**:

- Properties: Licorice root has anti-inflammatory, expectorant, and immune-enhancing properties. It's used to soothe sore throats, reduce coughing, and support adrenal health.

- Traditional Use: Licorice root has been used for centuries in traditional medicine to treat various ailments, including respiratory infections, digestive issues, and adrenal fatigue.

- Modern Applications: Licorice root supplements are commonly used to alleviate symptoms of respiratory infections, including sore throat, cough, and bronchitis. It's also used to support adrenal health and reduce inflammation in conditions like gastritis and peptic ulcers.

20. **Rhodiola (Rhodiola rosea):**

- Properties: Rhodiola is an adaptogenic herb known for its stress-reducing, energy-enhancing, and cognitive-boosting properties. It helps the body adapt to stress and improve mental and physical performance.

- Traditional Use: Rhodiola has been used for centuries in traditional medicine, particularly in Siberia and Scandinavia, to increase stamina, reduce fatigue, and enhance resilience to stress.

- Modern Applications: Rhodiola supplements are commonly used to reduce stress, improve mood, and increase energy levels. It's also used to enhance cognitive function, improve exercise performance, and alleviate symptoms of depression and anxiety.

Health Benefits and Uses:

1. Ginseng:

- Health Benefits: Ginseng is known for its adaptogenic properties, which help the body cope with stress and promote overall well-being. It boosts the immune system, enhances cognitive function, improves energy levels, and supports cardiovascular health.

- Uses: Ginseng is used to combat fatigue, enhance mental clarity and focus, improve physical endurance, and support immune function. It's available in various forms such as capsules, extracts, teas, and powders.

2. Turmeric:

- Health Benefits: Turmeric contains curcumin, a compound with powerful anti-inflammatory and antioxidant properties. It helps reduce inflammation, alleviate pain, support joint health, improve digestion, and boost cognitive function.

- Uses: Turmeric is used to manage conditions like arthritis, inflammatory bowel disease, and metabolic syndrome. It's consumed as a spice in cooking, taken as a supplement, or used topically in skincare products.

3. Echinacea:

- Health Benefits: Echinacea boosts the immune system and helps the body fight off infections, particularly respiratory infections like the common cold and flu. It also has anti-inflammatory and antiviral properties.

- Uses: Echinacea is commonly used as a preventative measure against colds and flu. It's taken at the onset of illness to reduce the severity and duration of symptoms. Echinacea supplements are available in various forms such as capsules, tinctures, and teas.

4. Ginkgo:

- Health Benefits: Ginkgo improves blood circulation to the brain, enhancing cognitive function, memory, and concentration. It also has antioxidant and anti-inflammatory effects, supporting cardiovascular health and reducing symptoms of conditions like Alzheimer's disease and vascular dementia.

- Uses: Ginkgo is used to support cognitive health, particularly in older adults experiencing age-related cognitive decline. It's available in supplements derived from ginkgo leaf extracts.

5. St. John's Wort:

- Health Benefits: St. John's Wort is primarily used as a natural antidepressant, helping regulate mood and alleviate symptoms of mild to moderate depression. It also has anti-inflammatory and wound-healing properties.

- Uses: St. John's Wort supplements are used to improve symptoms of depression and anxiety. It's available in various forms such as capsules, tablets, tinctures, and teas. It's important to use caution when taking St. John's Wort, as it can interact with certain medications.

6. **Garlic:**

- Health Benefits: Garlic has antimicrobial, antiviral, and immune-boosting properties. It supports cardiovascular health by lowering blood pressure and cholesterol levels. It also has anti-inflammatory effects.

- Uses: Garlic is consumed as a culinary ingredient and taken as a supplement to support immune function, cardiovascular health, and reduce the risk of certain infections. It's available in various forms such as capsules, extracts, and oils.

7. **Ginger:**

- Health Benefits: Ginger has anti-inflammatory, digestive, and anti-nausea properties. It helps alleviate digestive issues, reduce inflammation, relieve nausea, and improve circulation.

- Uses: Ginger is used to alleviate nausea, motion sickness, and morning sickness during pregnancy. It's also used to relieve pain and inflammation associated with conditions like osteoarthritis and menstrual cramps. Ginger can be consumed fresh, dried, as a tea, or in supplement form.

8. **Valerian:**

- Health Benefits: Valerian has sedative and anxiolytic properties, promoting relaxation and improving sleep quality. It's used to reduce anxiety, alleviate insomnia, and calm the nervous system.

- Uses: Valerian supplements are commonly used as a natural sleep aid and to reduce symptoms of anxiety and stress. It's available in various forms such as capsules, tablets, tinctures, and teas. It's often used in combination with other calming herbs for enhanced effects.

9. Chamomile:

- Health Benefits: Chamomile has calming, anti-inflammatory, and antioxidant properties. It helps promote relaxation, improve sleep quality, soothe digestive issues, and support skin health.

- Uses: Chamomile tea is popular for promoting relaxation, reducing anxiety, and improving sleep. It's also used to alleviate digestive discomfort, such as indigestion and bloating. Chamomile essential oil is used topically to soothe skin irritations and promote wound healing.

10. **Peppermint:**

- Health Benefits: Peppermint has digestive, analgesic, and antimicrobial properties. It helps relieve indigestion, reduce pain and inflammation, alleviate nausea, and support respiratory health.

- Uses: Peppermint tea is commonly used to alleviate digestive discomfort, including indigestion and bloating. Peppermint oil is used topically to relieve headaches, muscle pain, and itching. It's also used in aromatherapy to promote mental clarity and reduce nausea.

11. **Lavender:**

- Health Benefits: Lavender has calming, sedative, and analgesic properties. It helps reduce anxiety, promote relaxation, improve sleep quality, soothe skin irritations, and alleviate headaches.

- Uses: Lavender essential oil is used in aromatherapy to reduce stress, anxiety, and insomnia. It can be applied topically to soothe insect bites, burns, and skin irritations. Lavender tea is consumed to promote relaxation and relieve headaches.

12. **Aloe Vera:**

- Health Benefits: Aloe vera has anti-inflammatory, antimicrobial, and wound-healing properties. It helps soothe sunburns, promote wound healing, moisturize the skin, and support digestive health.

- Uses: Aloe vera gel is applied topically to soothe sunburns, insect bites, and various skin irritations. Aloe vera juice or supplements are consumed to support digestive health, alleviate constipation, and promote overall well-being.

13. Ashwagandha:

- Health Benefits: Ashwagandha is an adaptogenic herb with stress-relieving, immune-enhancing, and rejuvenating properties. It helps reduce stress, improve energy levels, support adrenal health, and enhance cognitive function.

- Uses: Ashwagandha supplements are used to combat stress, fatigue, and anxiety. It's also taken to support immune function, improve cognitive performance, and enhance physical endurance.

14. Holy Basil (Tulsi):

- Health Benefits: Holy Basil has adaptogenic, antioxidant, and anti-inflammatory properties. It helps reduce stress, support immune function, improve respiratory health, and promote overall well-being.

- Uses: Holy Basil tea is consumed to reduce stress, promote relaxation, and support immune function. It's also used in Ayurvedic medicine to alleviate respiratory issues, such as coughs and colds.

15. Milk Thistle:

- Health Benefits: Milk Thistle contains silymarin, which has hepatoprotective properties. It supports liver health, detoxification, and regeneration, and may help reduce liver damage caused by toxins or diseases.

- Uses: Milk Thistle supplements are commonly used to support liver health and detoxification. It's often used by individuals with liver conditions or those exposed to toxins, such as alcohol or environmental pollutants.

16. **Black Cohosh:**

- Health Benefits: Black Cohosh has hormone-balancing properties, particularly in women. It helps alleviate symptoms of menopause, such as hot flashes, mood swings, and sleep disturbances.

- Uses: Black Cohosh supplements are used to relieve symptoms of menopause and regulate menstrual cycles. It's also used to reduce symptoms of premenstrual syndrome (PMS) and support reproductive health.

17. **Saw Palmetto:**

- Health Benefits: Saw Palmetto supports prostate health and urinary function in men.

It helps reduce symptoms of benign prostatic hyperplasia (BPH), such as urinary frequency, urgency, and nocturia.

- Uses: Saw Palmetto supplements are commonly used by men to alleviate symptoms of BPH and support prostate health. It may also help improve urinary function and reduce inflammation in the urinary tract.

18. **Nettle:**

- Health Benefits: Nettle has anti-inflammatory, diuretic, and immune-modulating properties. It helps alleviate symptoms of allergies, arthritis, and urinary tract infections.

- Uses: Nettle supplements are used to reduce symptoms of allergic rhinitis (hay fever), arthritis, and urinary tract infections. It's also consumed as a tea to support overall health and well-being.

19. **Licorice Root:**

- Health Benefits: Licorice root has anti-inflammatory, expectorant, and immune-enhancing properties. It helps soothe sore throats, reduce coughing, support adrenal health, and reduce inflammation in the digestive tract.

- Uses: Licorice root supplements are used to alleviate symptoms of respiratory infections, sore throats, and coughs. It's also used to support adrenal health and reduce inflammation in conditions like gastritis and peptic ulcers.

20. **Rhodiola:**

- Health Benefits: Rhodiola is an adaptogenic herb with stress-reducing, energy-enhancing, and cognitive-boosting properties. It helps improve stress resilience, increase energy levels, enhance cognitive function, and alleviate symptoms of depression and anxiety.

- Uses: Rhodiola supplements are used to combat stress, fatigue, and mental fog. It's often taken to improve mood, increase physical endurance, and enhance cognitive performance.

CONCLUSION

Culinary Uses of Medicinal Herbs

Culinary uses of medicinal herbs involve incorporating various herbs into everyday cooking to enhance flavor and provide potential health benefits. Throughout history, different cultures worldwide have utilized herbs not only for their medicinal properties but also for their aromatic and flavor-enhancing qualities in culinary practices. Here's a breakdown of the topic:

- Historical Context: Since ancient times, humans have recognized the therapeutic properties of herbs. Culinary herbs were often used not just to add taste to food but also for their health benefits.

- Selection of Herbs: Certain culinary herbs have been found to possess medicinal properties. Examples include basil, oregano, rosemary, thyme, sage, mint, and parsley, among others.

- Nutritional Benefits: Many culinary herbs are rich in essential vitamins, minerals, and antioxidants, which can contribute to overall health and well-being. For instance, basil contains vitamins A and K, while parsley is a good source of vitamin C.

- Flavor Enhancement: Culinary herbs add depth and complexity to dishes, enhancing the overall taste experience. They can be used fresh or dried, depending on the recipe and personal preference.

- Health Benefits: Incorporating medicinal herbs into everyday cooking can provide various health benefits, such as improved digestion, immune support, and inflammation reduction.

- Integration into Daily Meals: Culinary herbs can be incorporated into a wide range of dishes, including soups, salads, sauces, marinades, and main courses. Experimenting with different herbs can lead to creative and delicious culinary experiences.

- Cultural Significance: Culinary herbs hold cultural significance in many societies. Traditional dishes often feature specific herbs that are deeply rooted in culinary heritage.

- Growing Your Own Herbs: Growing herbs at home is a sustainable and cost-effective way to ensure a fresh supply of culinary herbs. Whether in a garden, on a windowsill, or in pots, herbs can thrive with minimal care.

- Cooking Techniques: Different cooking techniques, such as sautéing, roasting, and simmering, can help release the flavors and medicinal compounds present in herbs, making them more bioavailable.

Herbal Teas, Salves, and Balms:

Herbal teas, salves, and balms are traditional preparations that harness the healing properties of medicinal herbs. These remedies have been used for centuries to address various health concerns and promote overall well-being. Here's a detailed overview:

- Herbal Teas:

- Herbal teas, also known as tisanes, are infusions made by steeping herbs, flowers, roots, or spices in hot water.

- Each herb offers unique medicinal properties that can address specific health issues, such as chamomile for relaxation, peppermint for digestion, and ginger for nausea.

- Herbal teas are easy to prepare at home and can be consumed hot or cold, depending on preference and the desired effect.

- Regular consumption of herbal teas can support hydration, relaxation, digestion, and immune function.

- Salves:

- Herbal salves are topical ointments made by infusing herbs into carrier oils and combining them with beeswax or another solidifying agent.

- Salves are commonly used to soothe skin irritations, reduce inflammation, and promote healing.

- Common herbs used in salves include calendula, lavender, comfrey, plantain, and chamomile, each offering unique skin-nourishing properties.

- Salves can be applied directly to the affected area and are gentle enough for everyday use.

- Balms:

- Herbal balms are similar to salves but often have a thicker consistency and may contain additional ingredients like essential oils for fragrance or enhanced therapeutic effects.

- Balms are versatile and can be used for a variety of purposes, including moisturizing dry skin, soothing sore muscles, and relieving minor burns or insect bites.

- Homemade balms allow for customization based on individual preferences and specific health needs.

- Like salves, balms are applied topically and provide targeted relief to the affected area.

- Preparation Techniques: Making herbal teas, salves, and balms typically involves simple preparation techniques that can be done at home with basic ingredients and equipment.

- Safety Considerations: While herbal remedies are generally considered safe, it's essential to research potential contraindications and consult with a healthcare professional, especially if you have pre-existing health conditions or are pregnant or nursing.

- Traditional Wisdom: Herbal teas, salves, and balms draw upon the traditional wisdom of herbal medicine passed down through generations. Incorporating these remedies into daily life connects us to our ancestors and the natural world.

9 798328 113595